FOAM ROLLING HANDBOOK

Beginners Guide To Self-Care With Foam Rollers

JESSE WILSON

Table of Contents

Introductory

Utilizing a foam roller to apply pressure to tense muscles and fascia is a common technique for self-myofascial release. Popular self-massage technique for reducing post-exercise soreness and accelerating recovery.

The foam roller is a cylindrical implement measuring between one and three feet in length and six inches in diameter. The application of body weight pressure and rolling movements can help relieve tension and trigger points in specific muscle groups and fascia (muscle connective tissue).

Foam rolling reduces muscle tension by applying repeated pressure to knots. As you roll over the foam roller, the compressive force applied to the muscle aides in the release of adhesions, the promotion of blood flow, and the activation of the stretch reflex. This procedure is advantageous for muscle recovery, flexibility, and pain.

Athletes, fitness enthusiasts, and regular people equally can relieve muscle tension and pain with foam rolling. In addition to being used alongside exercises, it can also be performed on its own.

When foam rolling, it is essential to exercise caution and operate within your own comfort zone. Unless directed at a tender location, such as a muscle knot, pain is not likely. If you experience sudden, severe pain, you should immediately seek medical attention.

Before beginning foam rolling, or if you have specific health issues or illnesses, it is recommended that you consult a medical professional or a certified fitness trainer to ensure appropriate form and technique.

CHAPTER ONE
Foam Rolling Benefits

Foam rolling may have multiple potential health benefits. The following are a few of the benefits that are frequently cited:

• By increasing blood flow to the muscles, foam rolling expedites recovery. If more oxygen and nutrients can be delivered to the muscles via enhanced circulation, there may be less muscle discomfort and a quicker recovery from exercise.

• Increased mobility and flexibility through the use of a foam roller to release tight muscles and fascia.

Due to its ability to increase flexibility and joint range of motion, it is frequently utilized by athletes and other individuals who wish to become more flexible.

• Foam rolling may alleviate muscle soreness and stiffness, thereby reducing discomfort. Trigger points, also known as knots, are excruciating, inflamed muscle areas that can be treated with this technique. By applying pressure to these locations, tension and pain can be relieved.

• Regular foam rolling has been demonstrated to improve athletic performance. It may improve movement efficacy and athletic ability by enhancing flexibility, range of motion, and loosening tight muscles.

• Foam kneading can be an effective method for preventing injuries. You can pinpoint tight or unbalanced muscle groups, allowing you to address the issue before it worsens. By keeping muscles mobile and functional, foam rolling may help athletes avoid injuries.

• Self-massage with a foam roller is a fantastic method to relieve stress and unwind after a long day. Thanks to the massage's rhythmic rolling movements and muscle pressure, the body can decompress and anxiety can be alleviated.

Numerous individuals have reported the benefits of foam rolling, but the underlying science is still in its infancy, and individual results may vary. Before commencing a new fitness or wellness routine, always pay attention to your body and consult a doctor if you have any concerns.

Use Of This Guidebook

Here are the measures you can take to make the most of this guide to foam rolling:

• Read up on the fundamentals of foam rolling to gain an understanding of the concept. Learn about foam rolling, its benefits, and why you should begin doing it.

• Consider what you hope to gain from foam rolling, and direct your efforts accordingly. Do you wish to expand your range of motion, reduce your risk of injury, accelerate your recuperation time, or target specific areas of tension?

Prior to foam rolling, it is crucial to determine your desired outcomes.

• Select a foam roller that meets your requirements. There are various diameters, densities, and surface textures of foam rollers. Foam rollers with a firmer density may provide a deeper tissue massage, but gentler rollers are more suitable for beginners or those with heightened sensitivity.

• When selecting a foam roller, it is important to consider how you will feel while using it and which areas you wish to target.

• In order to maximize the benefits of foam rolling and minimize the risk of injury, it is necessary to learn and practice proper technique.

• If you need assistance getting started, consult a fitness expert, physical therapist, or reliable resources such as instructional videos or literature on foam rolling. They are able to instruct you on how to perform all foam rolling exercises and stretches appropriately.

• Foam rolling is most effective following a brief bout of moderate aerobic activity or dynamic stretching to warm up the muscles. This increases circulation and prepares your muscles for foam rolling.

• Begin by concentrating on problem areas or specific muscle groups to maximize the effectiveness of your foam rolling session.

• Applying moderate pressure, roll the foam roller carefully over the affected area, pausing at any sore or tight spots. Maintain a steady and relaxed cadence, and avoid using excessive force or velocity.

- The level of pressure can be modified by adjusting your body weight and the amount of weight placed on the foam roller. Determine the best position and angle for working the desired musculature.

- Pay special attention to areas where you sense tension accumulating (trigger points and knots) and focus specifically on those areas. Consider applying constant pressure or gingerly rolling your sore areas for temporary relief.

- Consistency is the key to successful foam rolling. Include it as a preparation, cooldown, or solo activity in your regular fitness routine. Over time, consistent foam roller use can have positive effects.

• Listen closely to what your body has to say about foam rolling. It's normal to experience some discomfort, but you shouldn't subject yourself to anything unbearable. Adjust the pressure or technique if necessary, and if the discomfort persists, consult a physician.

• Keep in mind that this is merely an introduction; you should tailor your foam rolling routine to your specific requirements and consult experts as necessary.

• The study of the human organism is both fascinating and challenging. Consider the following if you wish to gain a deeper understanding of the human anatomy.

• Study anatomy to learn about the human body and how it is constructed. It is essential to study the body's systems and the organs, tissues, cells, and molecules that comprise them.

Included in this category are the skeleton, musculature, heart, lungs, digestive tract, nervous system, and endocrine glands.

• Physiology will teach you about the human body and how it functions. Physiology is the study of how the body's many interconnected systems govern and control vital processes such as breathing, ingesting, and moving.

• Educate Yourself on the Functions of the Body's Various Systems! Different systems serve distinct functions and interact in a variety of ways. If you want to understand how the body functions as a whole, you must study these systems.

- Learn about the smallest unit of existence by studying cells. Learn about the components and functions of cells, as well as the numerous types of cells that comprise the human body. Acquire knowledge of the metabolic, respiratory, and reproductive biological functions.

- Recognize the human body as a complex, interdependent system. It is typical for one region to be impacted by a change or dysfunction in another. For example, cardiovascular disease can impact other bodily functions.

• Investigate what it means to be healthy, what causes illness, and what factors can enhance your quality of life. This research focuses on common diseases, their causes, risk factors, preventative strategies, and treatment options.

• It is also essential to learn about the benefits of exercise, healthful eating, and stress reduction.

• Consider how the human organism develops and grows over time. Learn about the physical, mental, and emotional changes that occur over the course of a human's existence, from conception to old age.

Consider that your physical needs and capabilities will evolve as you progress through life.

• Review the most recent discoveries and studies in human biology and related disciplines. New research can revolutionize our understanding of the human body, leading to improved medical care and cutting-edge medical innovations.

• Consult specialists who have devoted their careers to studying and caring for the human body, such as physicians, nurses, and scientists. They are in a prime position to provide advice and answer any specific questions you may have.

• Recognize that your knowledge of the human organism is constantly expanding. Keep an open mind and actively seek out new data, resources, and learning experiences if you want to gain a deeper understanding of the topic and keep up with developments in the field.

Keep in mind that there is no single book that can teach you everything there is to know about the human body, as this topic encompasses so many disciplines.

You can learn even more about the human body by reading textbooks, trustworthy Internet resources, scientific journals, and engaging in in-depth conversations with experts.

CHAPTER TWO
How To Choose The Ideal Foam Roller

Several factors must be taken into account when selecting a foam roller to ensure that it suits your needs and preferences. The following are significant elements:

• Foam rollers are available in a broad range of densities, from very soft to quite stiff. Foam rollers with a gentler density are preferable for beginners, individuals with heightened sensitivity, and those seeking a more soothing massage. Deep tissue massage with a firm foam roller is more beneficial for those who prefer a lot of pressure or have particularly tight areas. When choosing the density of a foam roller, it is important to strike a balance between your comfort and intended difficulty.

• A diversity of foam rollers are available, each with its own length and size. Common dimensions range from one to three feet in length and six inches in diameter.

• Due to the additional surface area they provide, longer foam rollers are better adapted for planks and other exercises that require stability. Smaller, more portable foam rollers are ideal for travel and targeted muscle work. Choose a length and diameter that will facilitate rolling while allowing you to reach all trouble areas.

• A foam roller's surface may be smooth, textured, or adorned with designs such as ridges or knobs. Differently textured foam rollers are more stimulating to the senses and have a more profound massage effect.

People who desire more concentrated or intensive pressure in specific muscle areas may find them useful. Smooth foam rollers, on the other hand, provide a more uniform and consistent massage.

• When choosing the texture of a foam roller, it is important to consider both your personal preference and any areas of particular tension or sensitivity.

• The durability and quality of a foam roller should be determined by how long it lasts. High-density foam rollers are more resistant to fracturing or deforming over time. To determine the durability of the foam roller you're considering, read some reviews or recommendations.

• Consider how easily the foam roller can be moved and stored. If you want to transport it to the gym, travel with it, or store it in a small space, you can choose a small and lightweight foam roller. Some foam rollers are designed to collapse or have a porous center, making them more portable and convenient to store.

• Establish a budget for your foam roller. The price of a foam roller can differ greatly depending on its size, density, and quality. Consider what you desire, how frequently you will use it, and how much you are willing to spend.

• The purchase of a foam roller should be based on individual preference and feedback. Foam rollers are available in a wide range of sizes and shapes, so it's crucial to try out several models at a gym or seek advice from trainers, therapists, or other experienced users.

• By keeping these factors in mind, you will be able to locate a foam roller that suits your goals, preferences, and needs.

Preparing To Perform Some Foam Rolling

A few simple steps can make your foam rolling session more efficient and safer. Following is a primer to prepare you:

• Find a location that is spacious and free of distractions for your foam rolling exercises. Ensure that you have adequate space for movement.

• Dress adequately by selecting loose, comfortable garments that won't restrict your movement. This will allow you to apply the appropriate quantity of pressure while foam rolling. Do not limit your range of motion by wearing clothing that is too restrictive.

• To maximize the benefits of foam rolling, it is recommended to warm up your muscles beforehand. Spend five to ten minutes performing a moderate aerobic activity such as jogging, cycling, or dynamic stretching. This increases your central temperature, muscle blood flow, and readiness for foam rolling.

• Stay hydrated before commencing your foam rolling session and throughout the duration of the process. Hydration improves health in every aspect, from optimizing muscle function to lubricating tissues. Keep a bottle of water on board to drink during breaks whenever you feel thirsty.

• Determine attainable goals, such as which muscle groups or areas you hope to improve through foam rolling. Whether your objective is to strengthen your legs, back, hips, or shoulders, focusing on a specific area can help you organize your workout more effectively.

• Ensure that you have your foam roller and any other equipment or accessories, such as a mat or towel, before commencing. If you have all the necessary equipment on hand, your foam rolling session will go more smoothly.

• Familiarize yourself with the proper foam rolling techniques for the regions you intend to work on. If you want to ensure that you are performing the exercises properly, you should view instructional videos, read credible literature, or consult a fitness professional or physical therapist. When performed properly, the benefits can be amplified and injuries can be avoided.

• Make foam rolling more pleasurable by creating a relaxing environment. Reduce tension and anxiety by establishing a calming atmosphere with dim lighting and soft music.

• Prioritize your upcoming foam rolling session by relaxing and clearing your mind. Self-massage is most beneficial when performed in a calm and present-minded state.

Plan your foam rolling routine for post-exercise. After an exertion, static stretching, cool-down exercises, and the application of heat or cold therapy are all effective ways to promote muscle recovery. Creating a plan for what to do after your session will assist you in taking holistic care of yourself.

Consider that your needs and preferences may differ from those of others, and feel free to modify these preparation steps accordingly.

CHAPTER THREE
Methods For Foam Rolling

Foam rolling is intended to target specific muscle groups by applying pressure to the roller. Common foam rolling techniques for different body segments include:

1. The calves:

• Extend your legs and lie on the ground.

• Position the foam roller under your calf muscles.

• Raise yourself off the ground by your hips and support yourself with your palms.

• Apply moderate pressure as you roll from the ankle to the region just below the knee.

• If you feel a tender area, you should halt what you're doing and apply steady pressure for a few seconds before continuing.

2. The hamstrings:

• Position the foam roller in front of you and lie on it with your legs extended.

• For balance, lean back and place your palms on the ground.

• Cross one leg over the other to exercise the hamstrings individually.

• Concentrate on the back of your quadriceps as you roll from just above the knee to the base of your glutes.

• If there are tender spots, halt and apply constant pressure to them.

3. The quadriceps:

• Put the foam roller under your quadriceps while on your stomach.

• For support, lean on your forearms or extend your arms in front of you.

• To exercise the anterior thigh, roll from the pelvis to the region just above the knee.

• Apply more pressure to any sore or stiff areas for an extended period of time.

4. The IT sleeve:

• Place the foam roller under your pelvis while side-lying.

• Lengthen your lower leg and balance yourself on your forearm.

• Roll from the pelvis to the region above the knee.

- To alleviate IT band discomfort, slow down and apply gentle pressure to the affected areas.

- Stack one limb atop the other to exert greater force.

5. The Glutes:

- Cross one ankle over the opposite knee while seated on the foam roller.

- Lean forward over the crossed limb and roll the buttocks forward.

- Simply lean forward or backward to change the angle and focus on various regions.

• Maintain pressure on any knots to alleviate tension.

6. Middle rear:

• Place your upper back on the foam roller with your legs bent and your feet level on the floor.

• Maintain wide elbows while propping up your head with your palms.

• Roll from your upper back to your mid-back using your thighs as a lever.

• Stop when you reach a particularly sore or tight location

and allow the foam roller to do the work.

7. Lats:

• Position the foam roller beneath your armpit while lying on your side.

• Raise one hand with the palm facing upward to shoulder height.

• To target the side of the body, roll from just below the armpit to the lower ribcage.

• Shift your body position to modify the amount of strain on your lats.

It is essential to move slowly and deliberately while applying just enough pressure to feel a stretch or release without causing pain or distress when foam rolling. You can enhance the difficulty by repositioning your body or placing more weight on one leg. Pay close attention to your body and consult a physician if any concerns or symptoms persist.

Methods Of Rolling On Foam

Individuals have considerable latitude in determining the particulars of their foam rolling routines. Here are some examples of foam rolling workouts for different muscle groups.

Extensive Rolling of Foam:

1. The calves:

• Roll each calf for 30 to 60 seconds, paying particular attention to any tender areas.

2. The hamstrings:

• Roll each hamstring for one to two minutes from above the knee to the bottom of the buttocks.

3. The quadriceps:

• For one to two minutes, roll each thigh from the pelvis to the area just above the knee.

4. Use IT:

• Roll the IT band from the pelvis to the kneecap for one to two minutes per side.

5. The Glutes:

• Spend one to two minutes rolling each buttock, paying special attention to any knots or sore regions.

6. Upper Back:

• Roll the upper back for one to two minutes, concentrating on the space between the shoulder blades.

7. Lats:

• Beginning at the armpit and concluding at the lower ribs, roll the lats for one to two minutes on each side.

8. The chest:

• Position the foam roller under your mid-back and lie down on it.

• Extend your arms with your palms facing upward.

• Roll from your mid-back to your shoulder blades for a few minutes.

9. The shoulders:

• Lie on your back with the foam roller horizontally placed under your shoulders.

• Roll from the base of the skull to the summit of the skull for one to two minutes.

10. Proximal Back:

• Sit on the roller for one to two minutes while rolling from your lower back to your glutes.

11. Hips:

• Lie on your side with the foam roller horizontally under your hip.

• Spend one to two minutes rolling from the pelvis to the area just above the glutes on each side.

Remember that the duration and intensity of each rolling session should be tailored to your needs and preferences.

You can concentrate on tight or painful areas for a prolonged duration. Always take a few steady breaths before beginning to roll.

Particular Foam Rolling Workouts:

You can target specific areas, such as stiff hips or tense shoulders, while still incorporating full-body rolling. Here's an illustration:

1. Hips:

Roll the hips for two to three minutes, focusing on the buttocks and hip flexors.

2. Use IT:

• Roll the IT band on both sides for one to two minutes, beginning at the pelvis and ending at the kneecap.

3. The quadriceps:

• Roll each quadriceps (from the hip to just above the knee) for one to two minutes.

4. Upper Back:

• Spend two to three minutes rolling the upper back, paying special attention to the space between the shoulder blades.

5. The shoulders:

• Spend one to two minutes rolling each shoulder blade to the top.

6. The chest:

• Roll the torso for one to two minutes, focusing on the area between the midback and the shoulders.

7. The calves:

• Spend one to two minutes rolling each calf, paying special attention to any knots.

8. The hamstrings:

• 1-2 minutes should be spent rolling each hamstring from above the knee to the bottom of the buttocks.

Always ensure that the program is tailored to your needs and preferences for optimal results. If time is of the essence, you can shorten the duration of each continuous session or focus on the most urgent matters. One must be vigilant.

Effective Methods For Foam Rolling

Advanced foam rolling techniques allow for a more targeted release of muscle tension and a deeper penetration. If you want to take your foam rolling to the next level, consider the following techniques:

1. Activation of Trigger Points:

• Identify the muscle strain or trigger point causing the problem.

• Place the target area (the trigger point) of the roller directly on the foam roller.

- Apply constant pressure to the area for 20 to 30 seconds, or until you experience relief.

- Concentrate on the trigger point by sliding over it back and forth.

2. Stretch and secure:

- Target a specific muscle group and position the foam roller there.

- Apply firm pressure to the muscle to "pin" it to the roller.

- Maintain pressure on the muscle while performing a limb-bending or -straightening stretch.

• Pin and repeatedly stretch the muscle to achieve its maximum length.

3. To oscillate:

• Position the foam roller where you wish to exercise the muscles.

• Rather than rocking back and forth, maintain your weight firmly planted in a single location.

• To induce muscle vibrations or oscillations, make small, controlled movements.

• If you want to experience a sense of relief after 20 to 30 seconds, continue moving.

4. Surface Interactions:

• Align the surface of the roller with the muscle fibers.

• Apply side-to-side pressure to the muscle fibers.

• This technique can improve mobility by reducing adhesions and scar tissue.

5. Active Release Technique (ART):

• Incorporate the targeted muscle's active motions into your foam rolling routine.

• Perform joint or limb range-of-motion exercises while sliding over the muscle.

• It has been demonstrated that this method reduces muscular tension and increases both flexibility and range of motion.

6. Stretching Exercises for the Pelvic Floor:

• Perform a static stretch for the targeted muscle group.

• Stop stretching and immediately apply a foam roller to the muscle.

• Perform additional cycles of stretching and rolling.

• This technique combines stretching and foam rolling to enhance flexibility and muscle relaxation.

7. Spinal Mobilization

• While supporting your head and sacrum with your hands, position the foam roller vertically along your spine.

• Slowly massage the foam roller up and down your spine.

• Stop where you sense pain or tightness so that the foam roller can apply pressure and increase spinal mobility.

• Employ these cutting-edge techniques with caution and gradually increase pressure and intensity at first. If you experience severe pain or discomfort, reduce the pressure or discontinue the procedure. A fitness professional or physical therapist should be consulted before implementing advanced foam rolling techniques to ensure appropriate technique and safety.

CHAPTER FOUR
Personal Treatment, Including The Use Of Foam Rollers

Self-care practices such as foam rolling benefit not only the body, but also the mind and psyche. Here are some methods to incorporate foam rolling into your routine of self-care:

1. Foam rolling facilitates muscle recovery and reduces muscle discomfort by increasing blood flow and releasing tension in the muscles. Regular foam rolling can be used to address muscle imbalances, alleviate muscle tension, and increase flexibility.

2. Similar to a massage, foam rolling can have a soothing and relaxing effect on the body.

The stimulation of the parasympathetic nervous system results in decreased tension and increased relaxation. Including foam rolling in your self-care routine can help you relax, reduce tension, and feel better about yourself in general.

3. Foam rolling can help you develop a greater awareness of your body's needs and desires. By isolating specific muscle groups and knots, you can attain a heightened awareness of your body.

Understanding the strengths and weaknesses of your own body enables you to take command of your health by addressing any imbalances you may have.

4. Regular foam rolling reduces the risk of injury by increasing mobility and range of motion. By concentrating on specific areas of muscle rigidity, you can increase your overall muscular flexibility and reduce the likelihood of strains or imbalances that could result in injury.

Self-care practices such as foam rolling can help you avoid injuries and improve your performance over time.

5. Foam rolling is an excellent method to cultivate body awareness and mindfulness. You can strengthen your mind-body connection during foam rolling by focusing on the physical sensations and the respiration.

Mindfulness practice can help you become more in tune with your body, reduce stress, and expand your perspective.

6. As part of a self-care ritual, foam rolling can help you carve out time and concentrate on yourself. You can prioritize self-care and establish a healthy routine by reserving time for yourself each day, whether it's first thing in the morning or last thing at night. Including foam rolling as a regular component of your self-care regimen will assist you in developing a routine that nourishes your mind and body.

Always remember that self-care is an individual endeavor, and do whatever is most beneficial to you. Experiment to determine the foam rolling technique, duration, and frequency that works best for your body and overall self-care regimen.

How To Repair The Most Common Issues With Rolling Foam

In some instances, you may encounter difficulties when foam rolling. If you're experiencing difficulties with your foam roller, here are some common issues and their solutions:

1. Soreness or Discomfort:

• Use a gentler foam roller or cushion the area with a towel or yoga mat before you become accustomed to the pressure.

• As your muscles become accustomed to foam rolling, you can progressively increase the pressure.

• Do not roll directly on vulnerable skeletal structures or joints.

• If you are unable to roll the sore location directly, roll the muscles surrounding it.

2. Lack of stability or equilibrium:

• Foam rolling exercises are more effective when performed near to a wall or other stable surface for support and stability.

• As your stability improves, you can make larger movements.

• Use your abdominals and back to stabilize your body while foam rolling.

• If you need assistance learning proper form and equilibrium, consult a fitness professional or a physical therapist.

3. Unstable Foam Roller:

• If you are concerned about skidding, purchase a foam roller with a textured or nonslip surface.

• Use a non-slip mat or a sticky cloth to prevent the foam roller from moving around.

- When using a foam roller, it is essential to maintain a firm grip.

- If you have difficulty controlling a longer foam roller, consider switching to a shorter one.

4. The Expected Effect Is Absent:

- Modify your form or position so that you are strengthening the desired muscles.

- Determine the optimal foam rolling technique and angle through trial and error.

- Pay increased attention to these tense areas.

• Combine foam rolling with other stretching or mobility exercises to maximize its benefits.

5. Feeling Nausea or Vertigo:

• If you feel disoriented or nauseous while foam rolling, pause for a moment.

• Take placid, deep breaths while rolling to maintain stable oxygen levels.

• Consume copious amounts of water prior to and during the session.

- Seek medical care to rule out more severe conditions if symptoms persist.

Always monitor your body's response to foam rolling, and adjust your intensity, duration, and technique accordingly. If you have any concerns or persistent discomfort, consult your doctor or a certified fitness professional/physical therapist immediately.

The Conclusion

Foam rolling is an effective self-care technique with numerous favorable effects on health and well-being. By applying pressure with a foam roller, you can accelerate muscle repair, reduce muscle pain, increase your range of motion, and improve your overall health.

Choosing the right foam roller, gaining a comprehension of the body, and setting yourself up for success are essential for maximizing your foam rolling sessions. In addition, you can target specific areas and relieve muscular tension or stress by learning and practicing both basic and advanced foam rolling techniques.

You can enhance your physical and mental health by incorporating foam rolling into your routine of self-care. It helps with physical recovery, relieving tension, enhancing body awareness, reducing injury risk, and strengthening the mind-body connection.

Foam rolling can be challenging at first, but you can surmount any soreness, loss of balance, or slipping by altering your technique, equipment, or body posture. Common issues with foam rolling can be addressed to create a more enjoyable and effective routine.

It is essential to tailor your foam rolling program to your specific requirements, pay attention to your body, and consult with medical and fitness professionals as needed. Foam rolling can provide numerous health and relaxation advantages if performed regularly and deliberately.

THE END

www.ingramcontent.com/pod-product-compliance
Lightning Source LLC
Chambersburg PA
CBHW050748260726
48661CB00001B/471